CAYENNE PEPPER

MARIAN KIM

ISBN: 1508562210

ISBN-13: 978-1508562214

CONTENTS

MARIAN KIM

1

PROPERTIES

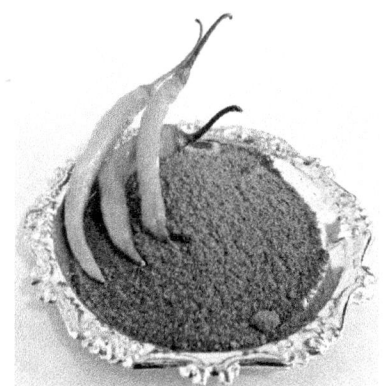

Scientific name: Capsicum annuum

Other names: African bird pepper, capsaicin, chili pepper, grains of paradise

Properties

The properties of cayenne pepper include:

Analgesic or pain relieving properties

Anti-aging properties

Anti-depressant properties

Anti-inflammatory

Antioxidant properties

Cancer fighting properties

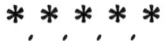

2

USES

Arthritis treatment

Cayenne pepper contains capsaicin which has pain relieving effects and is useful for the management of pain from rheumatoid arthritis and osteoarthritis.

This capsaicin causes local skin irritation which stimulates the nerves. This distracts the brain from the true source of the pain. Repeated application of capsaicin decreases the intensity of the pain stimuli or signal.

It is usually applied as a 0.025% capsaicin cream to treat arthritis pain four times a day.

Relieving pain

Cayenne pepper contains capsaicin which has pain relieving effects and is useful for relieving the pain caused by diabetic neuropathy (diabetes related nerve pains), HIV neuropathy, fibromyalgia, back pain, postherpetic neuralgia (shingles related pain), trigeminal neuralgia and cluster headaches. It is also used for psoriasis pain and for the mouth sores that develop after chemotherapy or radiotherapy treatment.

Depression treatment

Chilies have also been noted to elevate the mood by virtue of stimulating the TRPV1 pain receptor which results in the release of endorphins by the brain. These endorphins are the body's "feel good hormones" and they also result in the release of dopamine which is a mood elevator.

Cayenne improves digestion

When cayenne pepper is taken by mouth, the capsaicin can increase the secretion of digestive fluids in the stomach and thus aid food digestion. It also relieves intestinal gas, nausea, cramps and indigestion.

Diarrhea prevention

When cayenne pepper is taken by mouth, the capsaicin fights infection causing bacteria including those that cause diarrhea.

High blood pressure treatment

When cayenne pepper is taken by mouth, the capsaicin can help lower blood pressure since it dilates or expands the blood vessels.

High cholesterol treatment

Cayenne pepper is taken to lower high cholesterol levels.

Heart disease prevention

When cayenne pepper is taken by mouth, the capsaicin can prevent heart disease by lowering blood pressure and cholesterol levels as well as by preventing atherosclerosis or hardening of the arteries. It also improves poor circulation of blood and prevents excessive clotting of blood.

Nasal congestion relief

Cayenne relieves nasal congestion by shrinking the blood vessels in the nose and throat. This decongestant effect is useful for relieving the symptoms of colds and allergies.

Emphysema and bronchitis management

Cayenne pepper can be taken by mouth to prevent and treat emphysema since it thins the mucus and helps it move from the lungs.

Laryngitis relief

Cayenne pepper is used as a gargle to relive laryngitis.

Weight loss

Cayenne pepper contains a compound known as capsaicin which is useful for managing weight because it helps reduce caloric intake. It also increases the process of thermogenesis in the body in which fat is burnt to produce heat. Thermogenesis increases the metabolic rate of the body enabling it to burn more calories.

Diabetes management

A study published in the American Journal of Clinical Nutrition revealed that eating meals with generous amounts of pepper resulted in people with diabetes needing lower insulin doses after the meal to lower their blood glucose levels.

Muscle spasm relief

Cayenne pepper is applied on the skin to relieve muscle spasm.

Toothache relief

Cayenne pepper is use to relieve toothaches.

Seasickness relief

Cayenne pepper is used to relieve seasickness.

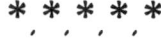

3

SAFETY PRECAUTIONS

1. Do not apply capsaicin cream to broken skin.

2. Cayenne pepper can cause skin irritation when applied to the skin.

3. Excessive consumption of cayenne pepper can cause ulcers.

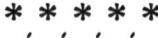

4

DRUG INTERACTIONS

1. Persons taking medications which slow blood clotting should not use/avoid cayenne pepper since it can also slow blood clotting. Medications which prevent blood from clotting include aspirin, clopidogrel (Plavix), dalteparin (Fragmin), enoxaparin (Lovenox), heparin, warfarin (Coumadin) and non-steroidal anti-inflammatory drugs (NSAIDS) like diclofenac and ibuprofen.

2. Persons taking theophylline should not use/avoid cayenne pepper since it can increase the side effects of theophylline.

5

COOKING TIPS

Flavor: Spicy hot

Goes well with: Meat dishes e.g. stews and soups, beans, chocolate desserts

Can be substituted with: Black pepper

To reduce the burning sensation, remove the seeds from the pepper before cooking or eating.

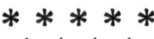

6

HERBAL RECIPES

Cayenne Tincture

Equipment

Glass jar with tight fitting lid

Dark tincture bottles

Cheesecloth

Labels

***

Ingredients

7 oz (200 gm) of cayenne pepper powder

30 oz (1 liter) of 80-100 proof vodka

***

Instructions

1. Fill 1/3 of the glass jar with the chopped herbs.

2. Add the vodka to completely fill the jar to the top.

3. Seal the jar and label it with the date of preparation and name of herb used.

4. Store the glass jar in a dark place for 6 weeks ensuring that you shake them weekly.

5. After 6 weeks strain out the herbs with a cheesecloth and pour the tincture into dark tincture bottles.

6. Label the tincture bottles with the date and name of herb used.

7. Store your herbal tinctures away from light and heat.

***

Tips

1. Pick herbs early in the morning just after the dew has dried.

2. You can leave the herbs in the alcohol for up to 6 months if you want to create very strong tinctures.

3. To make your tinctures doubly strong, you can pour the tincture after straining in step 5 above and store it for six more weeks.

4. Though the dose varies, a standard dose is 1 teaspoon diluted in water or tea and taken 1-3 times a day.

*****

Herb Infused Oil

Equipment
Double boiler

Large glass bowl

Sieve and cheesecloth

Sterilized dark jars

***

Ingredients
16 fl oz. (500 ml) pure vegetable oil such as sweet almond oil or sunflower oil

8 oz. (250 grams) cayenne pepper powder

***

Instructions
1. Place the cayenne pepper powder herbs and oil in the glass bowl ensuring that the oil covers the herbs. Simmer them in a double boiler for one hour at a temperature of around 120 degrees Fahrenheit (49 degrees Celsius). Do not let the oil and spice boil. You can repeat this step several times after letting the oils cool to create more concentrated spice infused oils. You can make your oils even more concentrated by adding more cayenne with each re-simmering.

2. Strain the mixture through the sieve and cheesecloth into a clean, dark jar ensuring you squeeze out as much oil as you can from the cayenne in the cheesecloth.

3. Label your jars with the manufacturing date, expiry date, herb and oils used.

4. Store your cayenne infused oils in a cool dark place or in the refrigerator and use them within 3 months.

*****

Cayenne Salve

Equipment

Double boiler

Large glass bowl

Sterilized dark jars or tins

***

Ingredients

8 oz. (250 ml or 1 cup) herb infused vegetable oil (see previous recipe)

1 oz. (30 grams) beeswax

50 drops (2.5 ml or ½ teaspoon) essential oils like lavender essential oil

***

Instructions

1. Place the beeswax and herb infused oil in the glass bowl and melt them in a double boiler.

2. Once melted remove from the heat source and add the essential oils drop by drop until you get your preferred scent.

3. Pour the melted oils into the storage jars or tins and allow to cool completely.

4. Store the salves in a cool dark place.

***

Tip

This cayenne salve is perfect for applying on aching joints.

*****

Cayenne Foot Soak

Equipment

Bowl

***

Ingredients

1 teaspoon cayenne pepper

1 cup of apple cider vinegar

***

Instructions

1. Mix all the ingredients in a bowl.

2. To use, soak your feet in it.

***

Tip

This cayenne foot soak is perfect for washing aching feet before applying the cayenne salve.

*****

Cayenne Butter

Equipment

Large glass bowl

Electric mixer or stick blender or wire whisk

Molds such as ice cube trays (optional)

***

Ingredients

½ cup butter

1 teaspoon cayenne pepper powder

***

Instructions

1. Place the butter in a warm place so that it can soften.

2. Put butter and cayenne in a large glass bowl and blend well until thoroughly mixed.

3. Refrigerate until it hardens. You can refrigerate it in molds or ice cube trays to give it a special shape.

*****

Cayenne Tea

Equipment

Kettle

Tea cup

***

Ingredients

1 teaspoon of cayenne powder

1 cup of boiling water

Honey to taste (optional)

***

Instructions

1. Put the herbs in a tea cup, add the boiling water and let it steep while covered for 10 -15 minutes.

3. Add honey (if desired) to suit your taste before drinking.

*****

Spicy Tea Spice Mix

Equipment

Jar with airtight lid

***

Ingredients

Cinnamon 4 tablespoons

Nutmeg 1 tablespoon

Cayenne pepper 1 tablespoon

Cardamom 1 tablespoon

***

Instructions

1. Mix all the ingredients and store in an air tight container away from heat, light and moisture.

2. To use steep 1 teaspoon of the mixture in 1 cup of boiling water for 15 minutes.

*****

Spicy Barbecue Rub

Equipment

Jar with airtight lid

***

Ingredients

Cayenne pepper 2 tablespoons

Garlic powder 2 tablespoons

Black pepper powder 1 teaspoon

Onion powder 1 teaspoon

Coriander powder 1 teaspoon

Cumin powder 1 teaspoon

Mustard seed powder 1 teaspoon

***

Instructions

1. Mix all the ingredients and store in an air tight container away from heat, light and moisture.

2. To use sprinkle on the meat to be barbecued.

*****

Spicy Chili Powder

Equipment

Jar with airtight lid

***

Ingredients

Cayenne pepper 4 tablespoons

Garlic powder 4 tablespoons

Black pepper powder 2 tablespoons

Onion powder 2 tablespoons

Paprika 2 tablespoons

***

Instructions

1. Mix all the ingredients and store in an air tight container away from heat, light and moisture.

2. To use sprinkle over the food.

###

ABOUT THE AUTHOR

Marian Kim is an experienced alternative medicine practitioner.

OTHER BOOKS BY THE AUTHOR

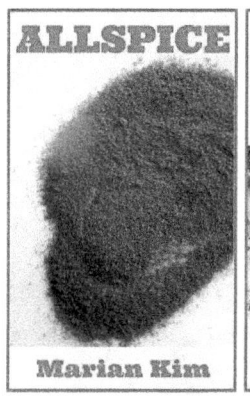

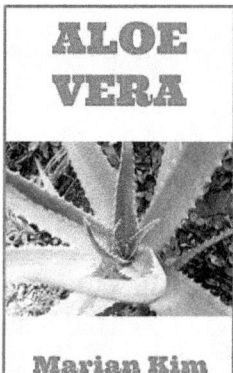

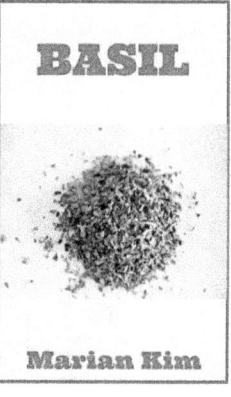

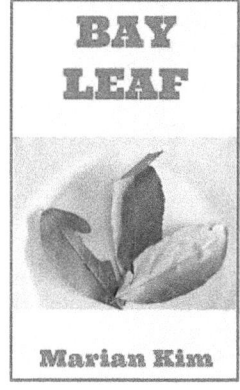

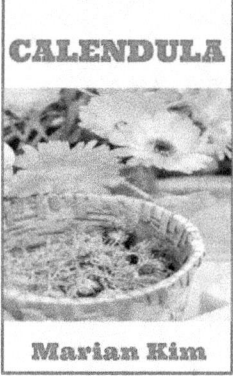

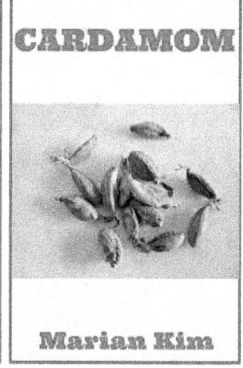

CAYENNE PEPPER

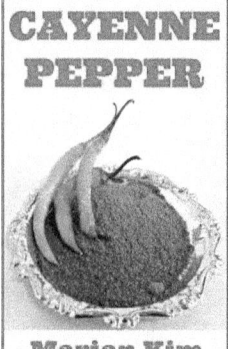

Marian Kim

CHAMOMILE

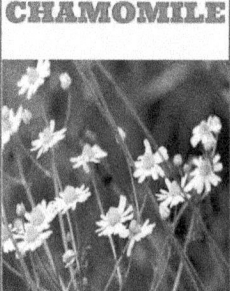

Marian Kim

CILANTRO & CORIANDER

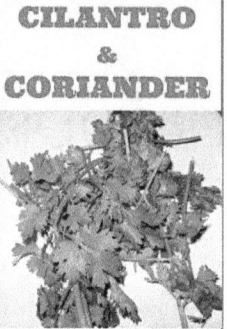

Marian Kim

CINNAMON

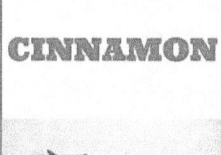
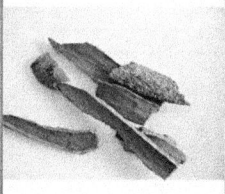

Marian Kim

CLOVES

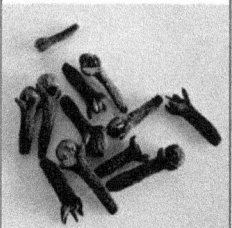

Marian Kim

CUMIN

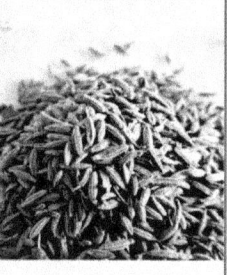

Marian Kim

DANDELION

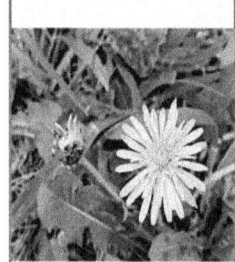

Marian Kim

DILL

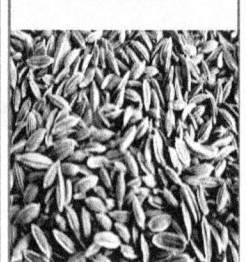

Marian Kim

ECHINACEA

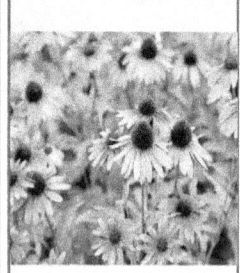

Marian Kim

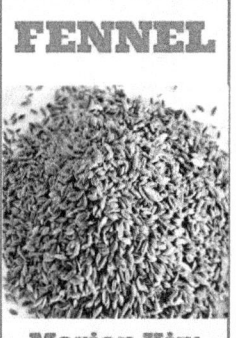

FENNEL

Marian Kim

FENUGREEK

Marian Kim

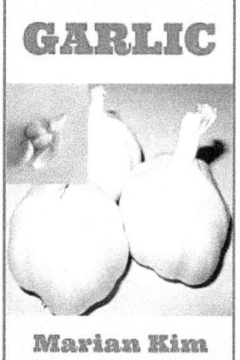

GARLIC

Marian Kim

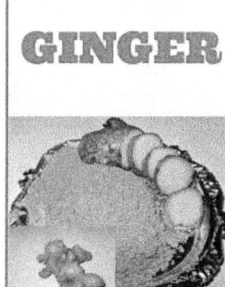

GINGER

Marian Kim

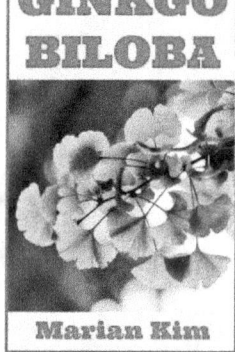

GINKGO BILOBA

Marian Kim

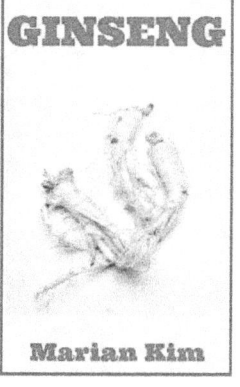

GINSENG

Marian Kim

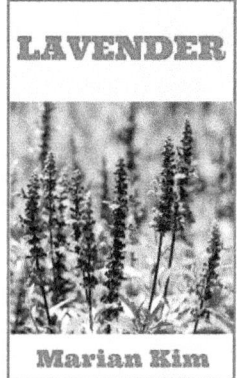

LAVENDER

Marian Kim

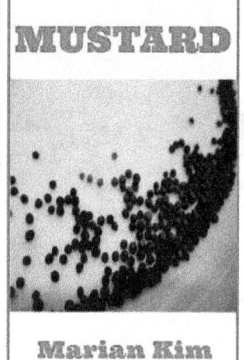

MUSTARD

Marian Kim

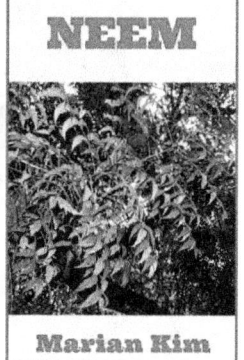

NEEM

Marian Kim

NUTMEG & MACE

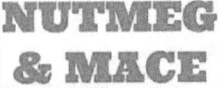
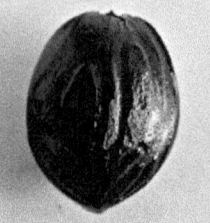

Marian Kim

OREGANO

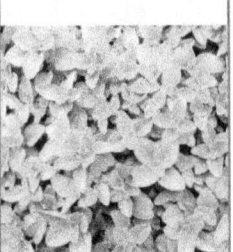

Marian Kim

PAPRIKA

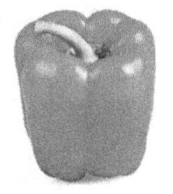

Marian Kim

PARSLEY

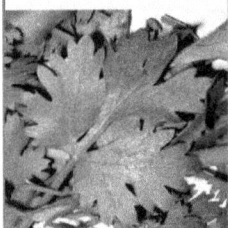

Marian Kim

BLACK & WHITE PEPPER

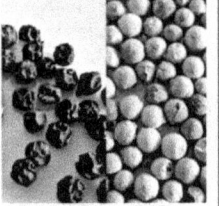

Marian Kim

PEPPERMINT

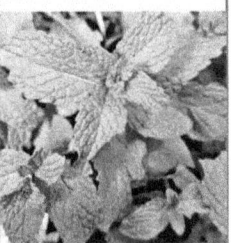

Marian Kim

ROSE HIPS

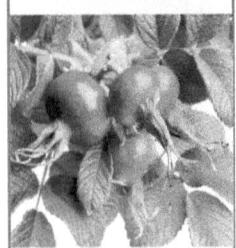

Marian Kim

ROSE PETALS

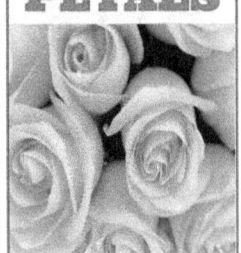

Marian Kim

ROSEMARY

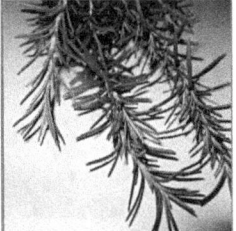

Marian Kim

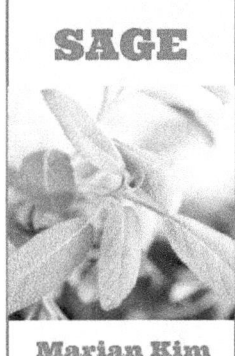

SAGE

Marian Kim

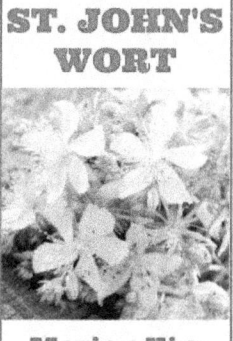

ST. JOHN'S WORT

Marian Kim

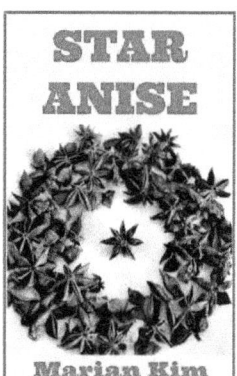

STAR ANISE

Marian Kim

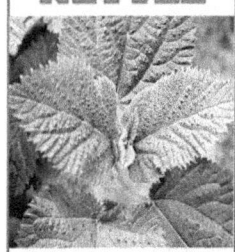

STINGING NETTLE

Marian Kim

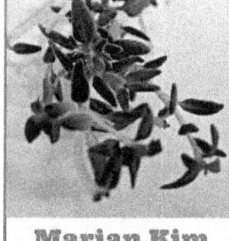

THYME

Marian Kim

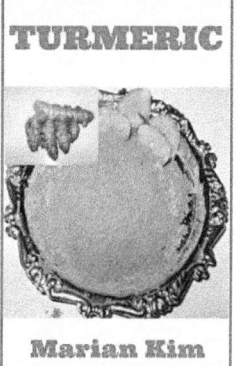

TURMERIC

Marian Kim

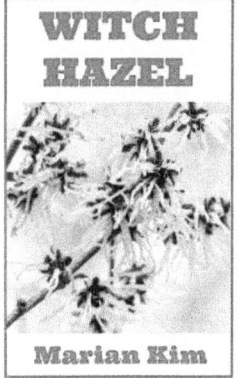

WITCH HAZEL

Marian Kim

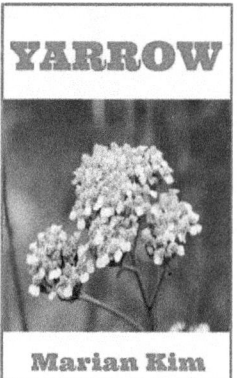

YARROW

Marian Kim

*****

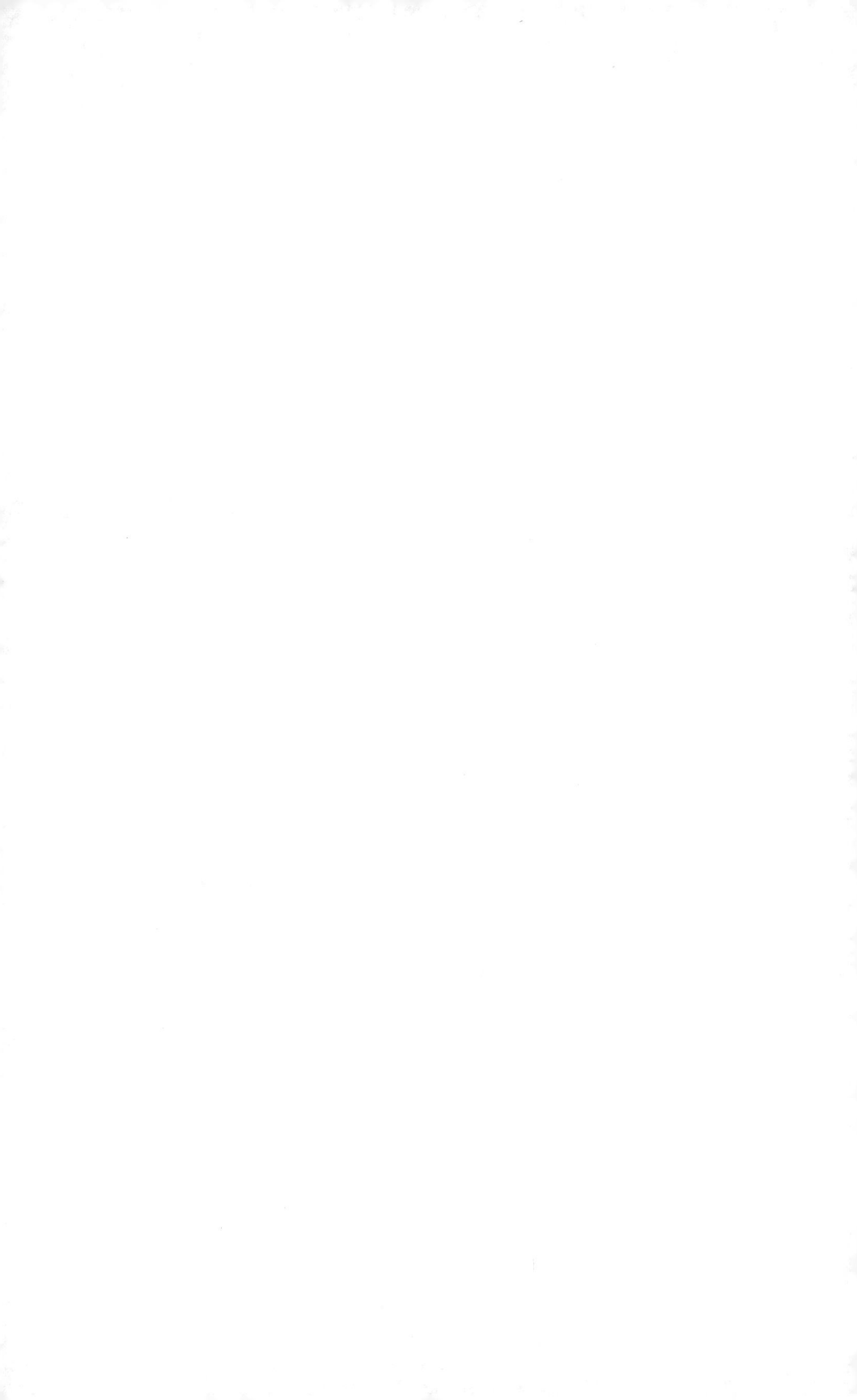